MENOPAUSE
MEANS . . .

MENOPAUSE MEANS . . .

NEVER HAVING TO SAY YOU'RE CHILLY

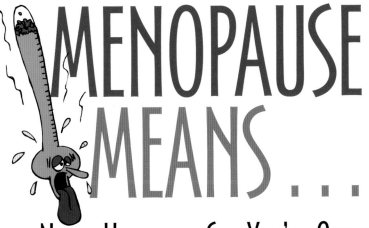

BY CATHY HAMILTON

Andrews McMeel
Publishing, LLC

Kansas City

07 08 09 10 11 SDB 10 9 8 7 6 5 4 3 2 1

ISBN-13: 978-0-7407-6861-3
ISBN-10: 0-7407-6861-1

Library of Congress Control Number: 2007921934

www.andrewsmcmeel.com
www.cathyhamilton.com

ATTENTION: SCHOOLS AND BUSINESSES
Andrews McMeel books are available at quantity discounts with bulk purchase for educational, business, or sales promotional use. For information, please write to: Special Sales Department, Andrews McMeel Publishing, LLC, 4520 Main Street, Kansas City, Missouri 64111.

1.
MENOPAUSE MEANS...

Never having to say you're chilly.

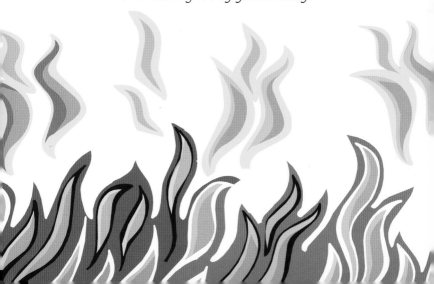

2.
MENOPAUSE MEANS...

Amending your personal definition of "crazy"
to exempt violent mood swings, spontaneous screaming,
and crying jags.

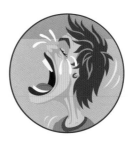

3.
MENOPAUSE MEANS...

Breaking down in sobs at the checkout counter when you realize you love Costco more than your husband.

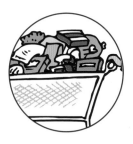

4.
MENOPAUSE MEANS…

Replacing your monthly period
with weekly chin-plucking sessions.

5.
MENOPAUSE MEANS...

Peppering your vocabulary with phrases like "Have I already told you . . . ?" "Did I reply to your e-mail?" and "Sorry I didn't return your call. Oh, I *did*?! What did I say?"

6.
MENOPAUSE MEANS...

Watching your family's facial expressions
change from amusement to terror
the moment you remove a burnt roast from the oven.

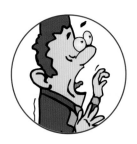

7.
MENOPAUSE MEANS...

Being so excited when you wake up
after getting five hours of uninterrupted sleep
that you can't fall back to sleep again.

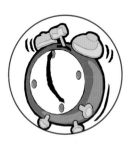

8.
MENOPAUSE MEANS...

Clearing your shelves of tampons, Midol,
and pads with wings only to replace them
with calcium supplements, progesterone cream,
and Preparation H.

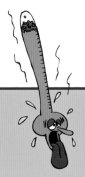

9.
MENOPAUSE MEANS...

Accepting the fact that your tube-top days
are definitely over.

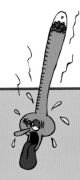

10.
MENOPAUSE MEANS...

Trading the fear of pregnancy for the greater fear of
a man with a Viagra prescription.

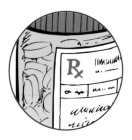

11.
MENOPAUSE MEANS...

Buying crossword puzzle and Sudoku books to fend off
Alzheimer's disease, then forgetting where you put them.

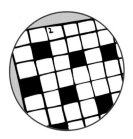

12.
MENOPAUSE MEANS...

Launching into a tirade over the horrible
customer service you received last Saturday,
then not being able to remember which store you
were in at the time or what you were buying.

(But the *point* is, whatever happened
to customer service?!)

13.
MENOPAUSE MEANS...

Asking the maitre d' in a five-star restaurant
to seat you at a table near a stiff draft,
preferably by the walk-in cooler.

14.
MENOPAUSE MEANS...

Immediately calculating the shortest distance to the
bathroom each time you set foot in a new place.

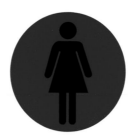

15.
MENOPAUSE MEANS...

Buying an assortment of fans in designer colors
for every room in the house.

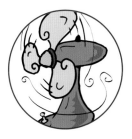

16.
MENOPAUSE MEANS...

Calling your own phone number every time important information pops into your head and leaving a message for yourself before you forget it.

17.
MENOPAUSE MEANS…

Lamenting the fact that the only freak flag you can fly anymore is the flesh under your arms.

18.
MENOPAUSE MEANS...

Reconsidering Arizona, Texas, or Florida for a cooler
retirement locale like Antarctica.

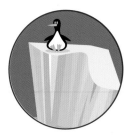

19.
MENOPAUSE MEANS...

Becoming intimately familiar with the shopping channel
hosts populating the airwaves at 3:30 a.m.

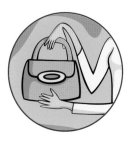

20.
MENOPAUSE MEANS...

Rifling through your purse for your car keys for
fifteen minutes before you realize you've left them
in your unlocked car with the engine running.

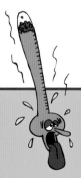

21.
MENOPAUSE MEANS...

Making Dr. Jekyll's alter ego, Mr. Hyde, look like a
well-adjusted model of stability by comparison.

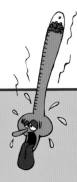

22.
MENOPAUSE MEANS...

Hanging a **CAUTION: FLAMMABLE** sign on your bedroom door.

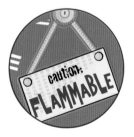

23.
MENOPAUSE MEANS...

Feeling like you've never been hotter
and not in the Paris Hilton way.

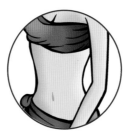

24.
MENOPAUSE MEANS...

Constantly being in the right place at the wrong time
and vice versa.

25.
MENOPAUSE MEANS...

Rethinking your former stand against face-lifts,
BOTOX, tummy tucks, and "anything that interferes
with the natural process of aging."

26.
MENOPAUSE MEANS . . .

Acquiring the uncanny ability to pop popcorn
by holding that little microwave pouch between your thighs.

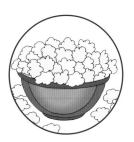

27.
MENOPAUSE MEANS...

Going from hysterical laughter to a flood of tears,
all in the time it takes to cycle through a traffic light.

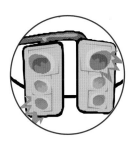

28.
MENOPAUSE MEANS...

Getting interrogated by the police after you've spent fifteen minutes trying to get into someone else's car.

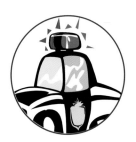

29.
MENOPAUSE MEANS...

Finding your reading glasses in the refrigerator
and not being at all surprised.

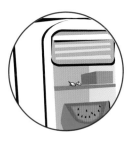

30.
MENOPAUSE MEANS...

Stepping outside in the dead of winter
and watching the steam rise off of your body.

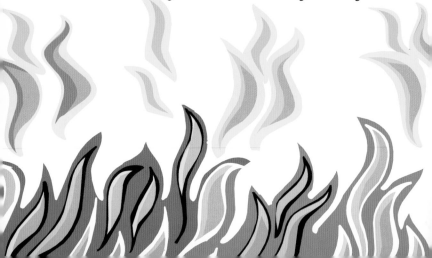

31.
MENOPAUSE MEANS...

Glancing down at your feet during a meeting with the boss
and realizing you're wearing two different shoes.

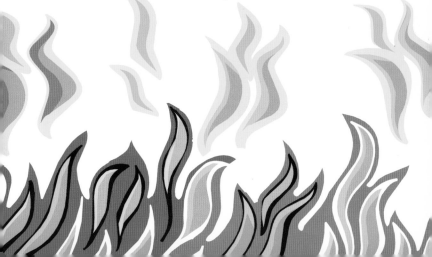

32.
MENOPAUSE MEANS...

Discovering in the dark recesses
of your medicine cabinet the bottles of gingko
and ginseng you bought a year ago
to prevent dementia.

33.
MENOPAUSE MEANS...

Not putting your summer clothes away in the winter
just in case you want to wear seersucker
on New Year's Eve.

34.
MENOPAUSE MEANS...

Always winning those nasty battles for thermostat control
because everyone else in your household
is too afraid to argue with you.

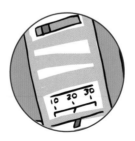

35.
MENOPAUSE MEANS...

Being on a first-name basis with your pharmacist,
electrolysis technician, and mobile locksmith.

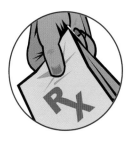

36.
MENOPAUSE MEANS...

Living in fear that every sneeze, cough, and hiccup
will cause you to pee in your pants.

37.
MENOPAUSE MEANS...

Buying moisturizer by the gallon and praying
it will last through the week.

38.
MENOPAUSE MEANS...

Using Rockette-like moves to kick your covers off
in the middle of the night when your body heat
reaches infernal levels.

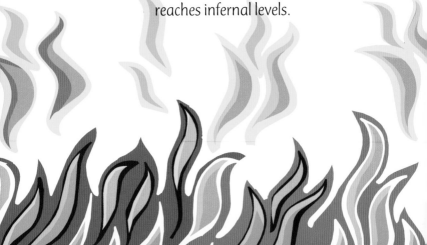

39.
MENOPAUSE MEANS…

Knowing that just one of your hot flashes
could generate enough power to heat your entire zip code.

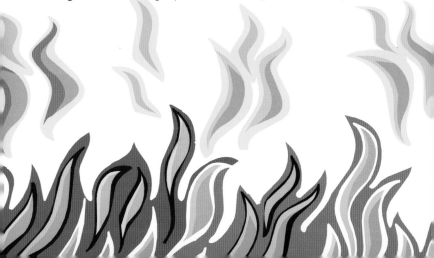

40.
MENOPAUSE MEANS...

Declaring a household state of emergency
when the air conditioner goes on the blink.

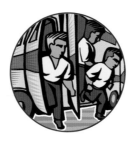

41.
MENOPAUSE MEANS...

Realizing, to your horror, that you have almost
as many whiskers as your seventeen-year-old son.

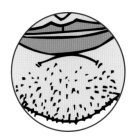

42.
MENOPAUSE MEANS . . .

Taking "hot and bothered" to a whole new level.

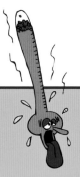

43.
MENOPAUSE MEANS...

Caving in and finally buying one of those
weekly pill dispenser boxes, then telling the clerk
it's for your elderly mother.

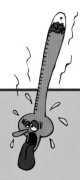

44.
MENOPAUSE MEANS...

Using the TV remote to **MUTE** your husband
and getting furious when it doesn't work.

45.
MENOPAUSE MEANS...

Trying to punch in so many PIN number combinations
at the ATM that the machine eats your card.

46.
MENOPAUSE MEANS…

Looking into the mirror and wondering what the heck your mother is doing standing in your bathroom.

47.
MENOPAUSE MEANS...

Having your *kids* ask *you*, "Do you have to use the bathroom before we go?" prior to every road trip.

48.
MENOPAUSE MEANS...

Getting a phone call from the grocery store
saying you left your debit card on the counter
and a case of Depends in your cart.

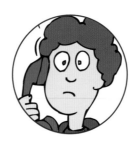

49.
MENOPAUSE MEANS...

Wearing that deer-in-the-headlights expression
when a friend approaches on the street and you
can't remember her name.

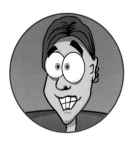

50.
MENOPAUSE MEANS...

Collapsing in tears when your GPS system
admonishes you for missing your turn.

51.
MENOPAUSE MEANS . . .

Breaking down during your annual mammogram
because it's the first time in years anyone has asked you
to take off your top.

52.
MENOPAUSE MEANS . . .

Thinking Lorena Bobbitt had the right idea, after all.

53.
MENOPAUSE MEANS...

Hanging a **NO RETURNS** sign on the door when your youngest child leaves for college.

54.
MENOPAUSE MEANS...

Having to take a sick day from work
after your first session with a personal trainer.

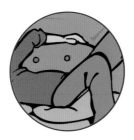

55.
MENOPAUSE MEANS...

Noticing that the hair from your legs seems to have migrated to your upper lip and chin.

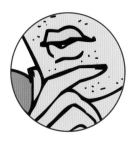

56.
MENOPAUSE MEANS...

Watching in horror as the gray hairs on your head start to resemble the coat of your wirehaired terrier.

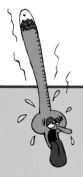

57.
MENOPAUSE MEANS...

Waking up one morning and discovering
all your pants are suddenly too tight in the waist
and too long in the legs.

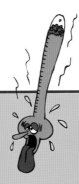

58.
MENOPAUSE MEANS...

Actually looking forward to your colonoscopy because at least you'll get good sleep afterward.

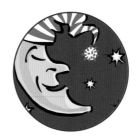

59.
MENOPAUSE MEANS...

Wandering through the grocery store aimlessly muttering,
"Now, what did I come in here for?"

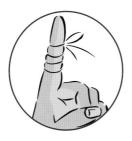

60.
MENOPAUSE MEANS...

Walking outside in your pajamas to get the paper
in the dead of winter and not even noticing
it's two degrees out.

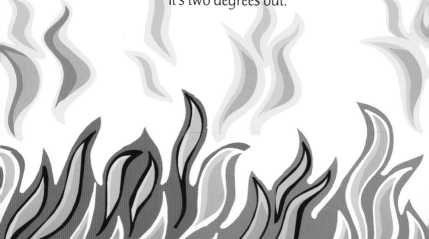

61.
MENOPAUSE MEANS...

Discovering curse words you never even knew
were in your vocabulary.

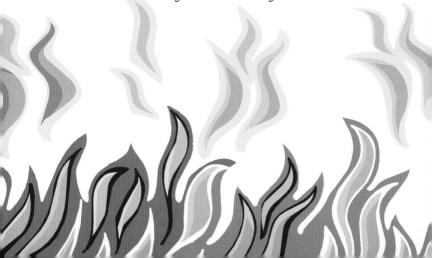

62.
MENOPAUSE MEANS . . .

Ordering your red wine with a side of ice
and applying the ice directly to your cheeks.

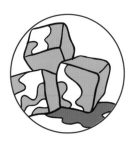

63.
MENOPAUSE MEANS . . .

Planning the perfect beach vacation to the
sunny shores of Nova Scotia.

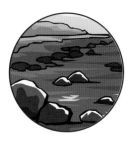

64.
MENOPAUSE MEANS...

Convincing yourself that choking the skinny little
college girl jogging on the next treadmill
would be justifiable homicide.

65.
MENOPAUSE MEANS...

The sign on the ladies' room door is enough to give you
an overpowering urge to "go."

66.
MENOPAUSE MEANS...

Answering the million-dollar question
every time you go out:
Do I wear the Spanx body-shaping underwear
and risk sweating profusely from my thighs all night
or stay cool with the cotton panties
and look like I'm six months pregnant?

67.
MENOPAUSE MEANS . . .

Having to go to the bathroom—
and "holding it" is no longer an option.

68.
MENOPAUSE MEANS . . .

Needing to count the remaining pills in your prescription bottle to determine whether you took your blood pressure medicine five minutes ago.

69.
MENOPAUSE MEANS...

Not really minding when you get the flu
and have to sleep on the bathroom floor
because at least it's cool down there.

70.
MENOPAUSE MEANS...

Babysitting your two-year-old potty-training grandson and
feeling like you have to go every two minutes, like he does.

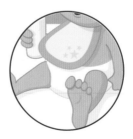

71.
MENOPAUSE MEANS...

Working hard to expand your mind
while your waist expands without a bit of effort.

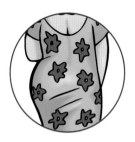

72.
MENOPAUSE MEANS...

Avoiding all sources of natural gas
and **CAUTION: EXPLOSIVES** signs
for fear you might spontaneously combust.

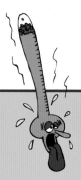

73.
MENOPAUSE MEANS...

Repeatedly hitting the elevator alarm button in a panic
and realizing, ten minutes later, you forgot
to push the button for your floor.

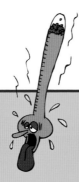

74.
MENOPAUSE MEANS...

Watching a steamy sex scene on TV
while the only thought going through your mind is,
"Did I remember to take the sheets out of the dryer?"

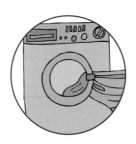

75.
MENOPAUSE MEANS...

Hanging your head out the car window like the family dog
when you need a "little air."

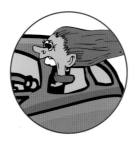

76.
MENOPAUSE MEANS...

Threatening the mail carrier with his life if he ever places
another Victoria's Secret catalogue in your mailbox.

77.
MENOPAUSE MEANS . . .

Getting comfortable with the fact that your
twenty-four-inch waist is a thing of the past
(if it was ever twenty-four inches to begin with).

78.
MENOPAUSE MEANS...

Changing your morning beverage from a
double-mocha espresso to a sugar-free decaf latte
with double soy.

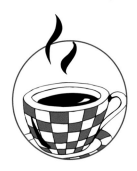

79.
MENOPAUSE MEANS...

Not knowing whether to laugh or cry
when the doctor tells you your bad cholesterol is good
and your good cholesterol is bad.

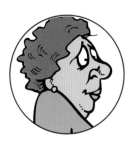

80.
MENOPAUSE MEANS…

Dinner conversation with the girls is no longer
about career moves and kids, but vaginal dryness
and diving libido levels.

81.
MENOPAUSE MEANS…

Developing a love-hate relationship with all of the
sleeveless clothes in your closet.

82.
MENOPAUSE MEANS...

Finding out a hair-trigger temper can be a good thing
when you're face-to-face with a crooked car mechanic.

83.
MENOPAUSE MEANS...

Thinking nothing of cutting in line and explaining
to the other women waiting for the restroom
that your incontinence problem is about to rear its
ugly head right there in the theater.

(Because it always works.)

84.
MENOPAUSE MEANS...

Being able to turn a door-to-door salesman into a
blubbering baby with just one look.

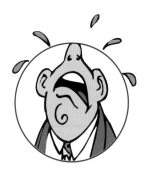

85.
MENOPAUSE MEANS...

Wondering how your biological clock can be speeding up
when your metabolism has slowed to a crawl.

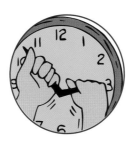

86.
MENOPAUSE MEANS...

Coming to the startling realization that you now prefer sleep to *sex*, food, *and* shopping.

87.
MENOPAUSE MEANS...

Lying awake at night wondering
if you actually swallowed that Lunesta an hour ago,
or if that was the night before.

88.
MENOPAUSE MEANS . . .

Burning more calories by tossing and turning in bed each night than you do during your waking day.

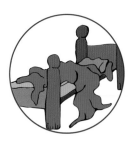

89.
MENOPAUSE MEANS...

Finally admitting you are powerless over chocolate
and not giving a damn anymore.

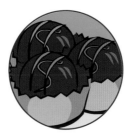

90.
MENOPAUSE MEANS...

Competing with your premenstrual teenage daughter
for "bitch of the week" honors and winning.

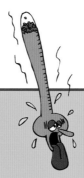

91.
MENOPAUSE MEANS...

Saying "hello" to elastic waistbands and "good-bye"
to elasticity in your skin.

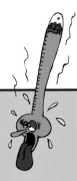

92.
MENOPAUSE MEANS...

Pining for the good ol' days of PMS when
water retention, crabbiness, and crying jags were only
a five-day-a-month occurrence.

93.
MENOPAUSE MEANS...

Constantly stroking your chin with your fingers
as if you're deep in thought (when, in reality,
you're just checking for new hairs).

94.
MENOPAUSE MEANS...

Getting an irresistible urge to strangle the clerk
behind the Clinique counter when the lipstick in the free gift
isn't your color.

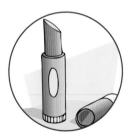

95.
MENOPAUSE MEANS...

Using the kitchen TV remote to turn off the microwave
and wondering why the stupid, blankety-blank thing
keeps beeping.

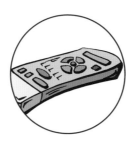

96.
MENOPAUSE MEANS…

Putting on a pair of shorts for the first time in the spring
and wondering what that extra fold is
hanging over your kneecaps.

97.
MENOPAUSE MEANS…

Worrying endlessly over things like trans fats,
bone density, polypeptides, antioxidants, triglycerides,
and the peritoneum, even though you don't really know
what any of those things are.

98.
MENOPAUSE MEANS...

Having a panic attack when the security guard won't let you bring hand lotion, Chap Stick, and bottled water with you onto the plane.

99.
MENOPAUSE MEANS...

Resorting to using breadcrumbs to find your way
back to your car in the mall parking lot.

100.
MENOPAUSE MEANS...

Never having to say you're sorry,
because you always have a built-in excuse.